Table of Contents

Leukemia is a cancer of the blood, characterized by the rapid growth of abnormal blood cells. This uncontrolled growth takes place in your bone marrow, where most of your body's blood is made. Leukemia cells are usually immature (still developing) white blood cells. The term leukemia comes from the Greek words for "white" (leukos) and "blood" (haima).

Unlike other cancers, leukemia doesn't generally form a mass (tumor) that shows up in imaging tests, such as X-rays or CT scans.

There are many types of leukemia. Some are more common in children, while others are more common in adults. Treatment depends on the type of leukemia and other factors.

BREAKFAST

1. Microwave Breakfast Burrito in a Mug (Mugrito)

Prep Time: 5 Minutes

Cook Time: 10 Minutes

Servings: 1

Ingredients

- 1 large 9 inch tortilla (flour or whole wheat)
- 2 eggs
- 2 tablespoons beans (pinto/black beans)
- 2 tablespoons cheddar cheese , grated
- 2 tablespoons scallions , chopped
- salt and pepper

Garnish

- salsa
- sour cream

Instructions

1. In a large microwavable mug press in a fresh tortilla. It will naturally fold into the shape of the mug and find its way.

2. Crack in your eggs and whisk up with a fork, taking care not to tear the tortilla.

3. Now add in your favorite burrito mixins like cheese, beans, and scallions. Season with salt and pepper and mix all together. Whatever ingredients you have to hand will work great.

4. Microwave for 1 minute 20 seconds. Check, and if the eggs are still liquid, cook for another 15 -20 seconds. Keep an eye during cooking so the eggs don't overheat. You don't want an egg-splosion in your microwave. The cook time is based on my 1200W microwave so yours might vary.

5. Once done, let it sit for 3 minutes to cool and serve with some sour cream and salsa on top. I like to eat a little out of the middles and then lift it out of the mug and roll it like a burrito.

Prep Time: 20 Minutes

Cook Time: 25 Minutes

Servings: 12

Ingredients

- 2 1/2 cups (12 1/2oz/355g) all-purpose flour
- 1/2 tablespoon baking powder
- 1 teaspoon salt
- 1/2 teaspoon onion powder
- 1 cup (8floz/225ml) milk
- 1 egg
- 1/2 cup (4oz/115g) sour cream
- 4 tablespoons (2oz/57g) butter, melted and cooled
- 4 green onions, thinly sliced
- 10 strips bacon, cooked until crisp then chopped
- 2 cups (8oz/225g) cheddar cheese, shredded
- 12 hard boiled eggs

Instructions

1. In a large bowl combine the flour, baking powder, salt and onion powder.

2. In a separate large jug combine the milk, egg, sour cream and melted butter until evenly combined.

3. Using a spatula, combine the wet and dry ingredients until a thick batter is formed. Lastly, fold in the bacon, green onions and cheddar cheese.

4. Preheat your oven to 375oF (190oC) then generously butter a 12 well muffin tin. Using 2 spoons drop heaped tablespoons of muffin batter into the bottom of each muffin. Next place 1 whole hard-boiled egg int the center of each muffin. Press down to ensure the egg is meeting the batter on the bottom of the tin.

5. Next, using the same two spoons drop heaped tablespoons of batter on top of each egg, using the spoons to push the batter down the sided of each muffin, this will ensure the egg is fully encased in batter. Repeat this process until all fo the muffins are completed.

6. Bake for 25 minutes until firm and golden brown on top. Allow to cool slightly before removing from the tin. Enjoy immediately.

7. Store in an airtight container in the refrigerator for up
    to 3 days.

Prep Time: 20 Minutes

Cook Time: 25 Minutes

Servings: 8

Ingredients

- 6 eggs
- 1¼ cup milk
- ¼ tsp salt
- Black pepper to taste
- 7 cups lightly packed baguette / french stick cut into 2 cm /
- 1 inch cubes (preferably slightly stale)
- 10 slices of bacon , cooked
- 2 cups grated cheddar cheese
- Parsley , finely chopped for garnish

Instructions

1. Whisk the eggs, milk, salt and pepper in a large bowl.
2. Place the bread in a large bowl and pour in the egg mixture, cheese and cooked bacon. Gently fold

together and set aside in the fridge for an hour or until all the egg is soaked into the bread. (I leave mine overnight in the fridge for really good soakage)

3. To Cook: Preheat oven to 350°F/180°C

4. Grease a 21cm/8″ springform cake tin. Pour the bread mixture into the cake tin, pat down the bread cubes to compress and scatter over a little more bacon and cheese if you have it. Cover loosely with foil.

5. Bake for 25 minutes, then remove the foil and bake for a further 10-15 minutes or until firm to touch in the middle. Allow to rest for 5 minutes before removing the springform and cutting into slices to serve.

6. Garnish with parsley and enjoy!

Prep Time: 25 Minutes

Cook Time: 45 Minutes

Servings: 10

Ingredients

Cinnamon Crumb Topping:

- 1/2 cup (2 ½oz/71g) all-purpose flour
- 1/3 cup (2 ½ oz/71g) sugar
- 1/4 cup (2oz/57g) butter, melted
- 1/2 teaspoon cinnamon
- Blueberry Muffins
- 2/3 cup (5oz/142g) sugar
- 1 egg
- 1/4 cup (2oz/57g) plain yogurt
- 1/2 cup (4floz/115ml) vegetable oil
- 1/3 cup (2 ½ floz/71ml) milk
- 1 teaspoon vanilla
- 1 1/4 cups (6 1/4oz/177g) all-purpose flour
- 1 teaspoon baking powder
- 1/4 teaspoon salt

- 1 cup (5oz/142g) blueberries, fresh or frozen

Instructions

1. Preheat the oven to 375°F (190°C). Place 9-10 muffin liners in a cupcake pan. Set aside while you make the cinnamon crumb topping.
2. Cinnamon Crumb Topping:
3. In a small bowl, whisk together flour, sugar, and cinnamon. Pour in the melted butter and stir with a fork until crumbly and place in the fridge while you make the muffin batter.

Blueberry Muffins:

1. In a medium bowl combine the sugar, egg, yogurt, oil, milk, and vanilla then whisk until well combined. Set aside.
2. In a separate large bowl stir together flour, baking powder, and salt.
3. Add the dry ingredients into the wet and whisk until just combined. Take care to not over mix, lumps are ok. Lastly, fold in the blueberries.
4. Evenly distribute the batter between the prepared muffin tin filling them almost to the top.

5. Remove the cinnamon crumb from the fridge and break it up into small chunks with a fork. Sprinkle the tops with the 1 generous tablespoon of crumb topping.

6. Bake muffins for about 40-45 minutes or until a toothpick inserted into the center of the muffins comes out clean.

7. Remove the muffins from the oven and allow to cool slightly before removing from the tin. Enjoy!

8. Store the muffins in an airtight container for up to 3 days. You can freeze the muffins in an air-tight container for up to 8 weeks.

Prep Time: 25 Minutes

Cook Time: 45 Minutes

Servings: 12

Ingredients

- 6 large eggs (at room temperature)
- 1 ¼ cups (10oz/284g) granulated sugar
- 1 cup (8floz/240ml) olive oil
- Zest and juice of 1 orange
- 2 cups (10oz/284g) all-purpose flour
- 4 teaspoons baking powder
- 1 teaspoon salt

Instructions

1. Preheat the oven to 350°F (180°C) and generously butter and flour a 12-cup (3.85 liters) capacity bundt pan. Set aside.
2. In a large bowl, whisk the eggs and sugar together, and then add the olive oil and orange zest, and juice. Whisk until combined.

3. In a separate mixing bowl, whisk together the flour, baking powder, and salt and then fold into the wet ingredients in three increments until just combined.

4. Pour the batter into the prepared pan and bake for 40-45 minutes, or until a wooden skewer inserted into the center comes out clean.

5. Let the cake cool in the pan for 10 minutes, and then invert it onto a wire rack to cool completely.

6. Dust with some powdered sugar before serving. Store leftovers in an airtight container at room temperature for up to 3 days, or in the freezer for up to 2 months.

Prep Time: 5 Minutes

Cook Time: 5 Minutes

Servings: 1

Ingredients

- 4 tablespoons all purpose flour
- 2 tablespoons sugar
- ⅛ teaspoon baking powder
- 1/16 teaspoon baking soda
- 3 tablespoons milk
- 1 tablespoon vegetable oil
- 1 tablespoon blueberries , fresh or frozen

Streusel topping

- 1 tablespoon (½ oz/15g) butter, cold
- 1½ tablespoons all purpose flour
- 1½ tablespoons brown sugar
- ¼ teaspoon vanilla extract

Instructions

1. In a microwave safe mug mix together the first 6 ingredients until smooth.
2. Mix in the blueberries.
3. In a small bowl, rub together the streusel ingredients with a fork until butter pieces resemble bread crumbs.
4. Sprinkle streusel on top of muffin batter, spreading out evenly across the surface.
5. Microwave for 1 minute or until it is firm to the touch on top (timing is based on my 1200W microwave so your timing might vary).
6. Enjoy immediately!

Prep Time: 15 Minutes

Cook Time: 35 Minutes

Servings: 1

Ingredients

Puff Pastry Crust

- 1 sheet puff pastry, homemade or store bough, trimmed to a 9 x 13 inch rectangle

Toppings:

- 4-6 eggs
- 1/2 cup cheddar cheese, grated
- 7 strips thick cut bacon, pre-cooked
- 1/2 cup cooked spinach, fresh or frozen
- 1 egg, lightly beaten

Instructions

1. First, preheat your oven to 400oF (200oC). Place your puff pastry in the Sweet Creations Nonstick Quarter Sheet Pan 9"x13"x1".

2. Using a small knife gently cut a 1" border around the edges of the puff pastry without cutting all the way though the pastry. This will help form the outer crust of the pastry after its blind baked.

3. Then, with a fork pierce the center a few times. This will prevent the middle from rising up too much during the blind baking.

4. Next blind bake the pastry by baking it on its own for 8-10 minutes. This will ensure the puff pastry is cooked through.

5. Remove from the oven and sprinkle the cheese over the middle. Then layer on the spinach and bacon, arranging in one even layer across the tart. Lastly, crack on the eggs leaving space between each one.

6. Bake for 12-15 minutes or until the white of the egg is fully cooked and the yellow of the egg is set on the outside but still a little runny. if you only like you eggs firm feel free to bake for a few minutes longer.

7. Allow to cool for a few minutes before cutting into individual portions with a knife or pizza cutter. Cover and store in the fridge for 1-2 days.

Prep Time: 15 Minutes

Cook Time: 35 Minutes

Servings: 1

Ingredients

Waffles:

- 3 cups all-purpose flour
- 1 Tablespoon baking powder
- 1 teaspoon baking soda
- 1 teaspoon salt
- ¼ cup sugar
- 2/3 cups canola oil
- 4 large eggs
- 2 teaspoons vanilla extract
- 2½ cups buttermilk
- Churro topping - Cinnamon Sugar
- ½ Cup of Sugar
- ¼ Cup ground Cinnamon
- ½ cup/50g Melted Butter
- Chocolate Ganache (Sauce)

- 8 ounces semisweet or bittersweet chocolate (we like 72 percent cacao)
- 1 cup heavy cream

Instructions

Waffle Batter

1. In a large bowl combine flour, baking powder, baking soda, salt and sugar.
2. In a jug, whisk together eggs, oil, buttermilk and vanilla extract.
3. Whisk to spell out W.A.F.F.L.E.S, or 7 times roughly. A few Lumps and bumps are all good. Just like pancake batter, they work themselves out while the batter rests
4. Refrigerate for 10-20 minutes and get working on your sauce and cinnamon sugar.

Chocolate Ganache (Sauce)

1. Heat the cream until it is about to boil, then turn it off
2. Pour over the chopped chocolate and whisk until smooth and shiny. Set aside until needed

Churro Topping

1. Melt the butter and set aside

2. Mix the cinnamon and sugar in a bowl together until well combined.

3. Cooking Waffles: pre-heat your waffle iron to medium heat. Grease with butter

4. Spoon the batter into a preheated waffle iron.

5. Cook the waffles until golden and crisp. (all waffle irons are different but roughly around 3-4 minutes)

6. TIP: Resist the urge to open the waffle iron while cooking so you don't let out all that lovely steam that will give you a chrisp, brown waffle

7. Once fully cooked immediately brush with melted butter and sprinkle over you cinnamon sugar. Turn over and do the same on the other side. Don't be shy with the cinnamon sugar, it's the best part.

8. Drizzle over the warm, rich chocolate sauce to get that full Churro experience. If you are feeling extra BOLD then finish with freshly whipped cream like I did!!

Prep Time: 25 Minutes

Cook Time: 45 Minutes

Servings: 10

Ingredients

Cinnamon Crumb Topping

- 1/2 cup (2 ½oz/71g) all-purpose flour
- 1/3 cup (2 ½ oz/71g) sugar
- 1/4 cup (2oz/57g) butter, melted
- 1/2 teaspoon cinnamon
- Blueberry Muffins
- 2/3 cup (5oz/142g) sugar
- 1 egg
- 1/4 cup (2oz/57g) plain yogurt
- 1/2 cup (4floz/115ml) vegetable oil
- 1/3 cup (2 ½ floz/71ml) milk
- 1 teaspoon vanilla
- 1 1/4 cups (6 1/4oz/177g) all-purpose flour
- 1 teaspoon baking powder
- 1/4 teaspoon salt

* 1 cup (5oz/142g) blueberries, fresh or frozen

Instructions

1. Preheat the oven to 375°F (190°C). Place 9-10 muffin liners in a cupcake pan. Set aside while you make the cinnamon crumb topping.
2. Cinnamon Crumb Topping:
3. In a small bowl, whisk together flour, sugar, and cinnamon. Pour in the melted butter and stir with a fork until crumbly and place in the fridge while you make the muffin batter.

Blueberry Muffins:

1. In a medium bowl combine the sugar, egg, yogurt, oil, milk, and vanilla then whisk until well combined. Set aside.
2. In a separate large bowl stir together flour, baking powder, and salt.
3. Add the dry ingredients into the wet and whisk until just combined. Take care to not over mix, lumps are ok. Lastly, fold in the blueberries.
4. Evenly distribute the batter between the prepared muffin tin filling them almost to the top.

5. Remove the cinnamon crumb from the fridge and break it up into small chunks with a fork. Sprinkle the tops with the 1 generous tablespoon of crumb topping.

6. Bake muffins for about 40-45 minutes or until a toothpick inserted into the center of the muffins comes out clean.

7. Remove the muffins from the oven and allow to cool slightly before removing from the tin. Enjoy!

8. Store the muffins in an airtight container for up to 3 days. You can freeze the muffins in an air-tight container for up to 8 weeks.

11. Cheesy Corn Fritters

Prep Time: 10 Minutes

Cook Time: 15 Minutes

Servings: 12

Ingredients

- 3 cups corn kernels, approximately 4 corn cobs
- ¼ cup cilantro, chopped
- ¼ cup green onion, chopped
- 1 jalapeno , deseeded, membranes removed, diced
- juice from 1/2 a lime, 1 tablespoon
- 1 cup all purpose flour
- 1 tsp baking powder
- ½ tsp salt
- ¼ tsp ground black pepper
- ¼ tsp chili powder
- 2 large eggs , beaten
- ¼ cup milk
- 1½ cup Monterey Jack Cheese, shredded
- 2 tbsp extra virgin olive oil

Instructions

1. Prepare Corn: Add the corn to a large bowl. If using fresh corn, cut all the kernels off the cob. If using canned or frozen check notes at bottom of recipe.
2. Add in the diced green cilantro, green onion, diced jalapeno, and squeeze in the lime juice from 1/2 a lime.
3. Mix Dry Ingredients: In a small bowl add the flour, baking powder, salt, black pepper, chili powder and stir to combine.
4. Combine: Pour the dry ingredients into the bowl with the corn. Stir to mix together.
5. Mix Batter: Pour in the beaten eggs, milk, and cheese. Stir to combine. Will be a thick batter.
6. Heat Oil: Heat a pan over medium high heat, add a drizzle of olive oil, we just need to coat the bottom of the pan.
7. Fry Fritters: Place a scoop of the corn fritter batter, about a 1/4 cup amount into the hot oil. Press the batter down to compact it, and press the sides in to help create a patty shape using a rubber spatula.
8. Let the batter cook in the oil for about 2-3 minutes, you will see the edges starting to turn golden. Then carefully flip using a spatula to cook the other side.

Once both sides are golden brown then remove from the pan and set on a tray lined with a paper towel to absorb any extra oil.

9. At this point you can sprinkle with any extra salt or pepper you may want. Serve warm.

Prep Time: 5 Minutes

Cook Time: 20 Minutes

Servings: 6

Ingredients

- 1 lb ground beef
- ½ yellow onion, diced
- 3 cloves garlic, minced
- 1 tsp salt
- 1 tsp cumin
- 1½ tsp chili powder
- ½ tsp black pepper
- 1 tsp dried oregano
- 1 (28 ounce can) crushed tomatoes
- 2 cups beef broth
- 1 (4 ounce can) diced green chiles
- 1 (15 ounce can) black beans , drained and rinsed
- 1 (15.25 ounce can) whole kernel golden sweet corn, or 1 and 1/2 cup frozen corn kernels

Toppings (Optional):

- cheddar cheese, shredded
- sour cream
- tortilla chips
- cilantro, diced

Instructions

1. Cook Ground Beef: Add the ground beef to a large pot, cook the meat over medium heat until mostly browned, add the diced onion and continue cooking, stirring occasionally until the meat is browned. Add in the minced garlic and cook for another 30 seconds.
2. Drain & Season: Drain the grease and return the pot to the stovetop. Add the seasonings (salt, cumin, chili powder, black pepper, oregano). Stir to combine.
3. Create Broth: Pour in the crushed tomatoes and beef broth, add in the black beans, green chiles and corn. Stir to combine.
4. Simmer: Bring soup to a simmer, cover and reduce heat to low. Let this cook for 10 minutes.
5. Serve: Top with shredded cheese, sour cream, diced cilantro, and tortilla chips.

Prep Time: 5 Minutes

Cook Time: 5 Minutes

Servings: 2

Ingredients

- 2 cups baby spinach, raw
- ¼ cup dried cranberries
- ¼ cup pecans, halved
- 2 tbsp feta cheese
- ½ granny smith apple , sliced
- ½ fuji apple , sliced
- 2 slices bacon , cooked and chopped

Maple Dijon Vinaigrette:

- 2 tbsp extra virgin olive oil
- 1 tbsp apple cider vinegar
- 1 tbsp maple syrup
- 1½ tsp dijon mustard
- salt & pepper to taste

Instructions

1. Make Dressing: Add all the ingredients for the maple dijon vinaigrette to a small mason jar. Shake to mix.
2. Layer Salad: Add the spinach to a medium size bowl or plate.
3. Top with dried cranberries, halved pecans, feta cheese, sliced apples, and cooked bacon.
4. Dress and Toss: Drizzle the salad dressing over the top of the salad, toss and serve.

Prep Time: 5 Minutes

Cook Time: 25 Minutes

Servings: 2

Ingredients

- 1 naan bread
- 1 tsp Organic Extra Virgin Olive Oil
- 1 clove garlic , minced
- 2 tbsp Organics hummus
- ¼ cup Organics Half and Half Salad Mix
- ¼ cup cherry tomatoes , halved
- ¼ cup Kalamata olives , halved
- 2 tbsp feta, crumbled
- Red onion , sliced
- ¼ cup garlic roasted chickpeas, directions below

Garlic Roasted Chickpeas:

- 1 (14 ounce) garbanzo beans, drained and rinsed
- ½ tbsp extra virgin olive oil
- ¼ tsp garlic powder
- ¼ tsp salt

Instructions

Garlic Roasted Chickpeas

1. Preheat oven to 425°F. Line a small baking sheet with parchment paper and set aside.
2. Rinse and drain the garbanzo beans. Spread out and pat dry with a paper towel. Remove any skins that are coming off. There's no need to remove them all.
3. Add beans to a small bowl or large resealable plastic bag.
4. Drizzle with Organics Extra Virgin Olive Oil. Sprinkle with garlic powder and salt. Shake or stir to combine.
5. Spread out on the small baking sheet. Keep them clustered together to help prevent burning, but keep them in a single layer to ensure crispness.
6. Bake for 25-30 minutes stirring every 10 minutes to ensure all sides are crisp and they don't burn.

Hummus Flat Bread Pizza

1. Preheat oven to 350°F. Lay the naan bread on a small baking sheet lined with parchment paper. Drizzle with 1 teaspoon
2. Organics Extra Virgin Olive Oil, brush to coat and then add the minced garlic. Heat for 10 minutes or until warmed through.

3. Spread with Organics Hummus. Layer with toppings.

4. Serve warm and enjoy.

Prep Time: 5 Minutes

Cook Time: 15 Minutes

Servings: 6

Ingredients

- 1 pound ground beef
- 1 tbsp Chili Powder
- ½ tsp Salt
- ¾ tsp Cumin
- ½ tsp Dried Oregano
- ¼ tsp Garlic Powder
- ¼ tsp Onion Powder
- 4 ounces tomato sauce
- 3 avocados halved
- 1 cup cheddar cheese, shredded
- ¼ cup cherry tomatoes , sliced
- ¼ cup lettuce , shredded

Additional Toppings:

- cilantro
- sour cream

Instructions

1. Add the ground beef to a medium size sauce pan. Cook over medium heat until browned.

2. Drain the grease and add the seasonings and the tomato sauce. Stir to combine. Cook for about 3-4 minutes.

3. Remove the pit from the halved avocados. Load the crater left from the pit with the taco meat. Top with cheese, tomatoes, lettuce, cilantro and sour cream.

4. If you want to make a larger area in the avocado for the toppings, spoon out some of the avocado and set aside to make guacamole! Then fill with toppings.

Prep Time: 20 Minutes

Cook Time: 0 Minutes

Servings: 2

Ingredients

Cilantro Lime Rice:

- 1/2 cup white rice
- 1 cup water
- 1/4 tsp lime juice
- 1 tsp cilantro, chopped
- pinch salt

Avocado:

- 1 medium ripe avocado
- 1/8 tsp lime juice
- Pinch salt

Spicy Mayo:

- 1/2 cup mayonnaise
- 1 tbsp sriracha, or less to taste
- 1/2 tsp chili oil

- 1 medium cucumber , peeled, chopped
- 1 (5 ounce) Can Chicken of the Sea Skinless & Boneless Pink Salmon
- 3 green onions , chopped

Instructions

1. Prepare the rice by cooking the white rice in the water according to the directions.
2. Once cooked and cooled add in the lime juice, cilantro and a pinch of salt to taste.
3. Mash the avocado in a small bowl and add the splash of lime juice, and pinch of salt. Stir to combine.
4. Prepare the spicy mayo by mixing the mayonnaise, sriracha, and chili oil together. Add less oil and/or sriracha to make it less spicy if needed. Stir to combine.
5. In a small bowl add the Chicken of the Sea® Skinless & Boneless Pink Salmon, add 1 tablespoon of the spicy mayo and stir to combine. Salt to taste if needed.
6. In a 1 cup measuring cup add the chopped cucumber, spread a layer of the mashed avocado. Press it down to ensure it is packed into the cup. Add a layer of the Chicken of the Sea Skinless & Boneless Pink Salmon

mixture, press down to ensure that it is packed. Then add the layer of the cilantro lime rice, press down to pack.

7. Run a butter knife along the inside of the cup. Turn the cup upside down carefully onto a flat surface and gently lift.

8. Sprinkle with green onion and drizzle with spicy mayo. Serve and enjoy!

Prep Time: 10 Minutes

Cook Time: 40 Minutes

Servings: 6

Ingredients

- 4-5 sweet potatoes, approximately 3 pounds
- 1/2 cup unsalted butter
- 1/3 cup light brown sugar
- 1/3 cup maple syrup
- 1 teaspoon ground cinnamon
- 1/2 teaspoon ground nutmeg
- 1/2 teaspoon ground ginger
- pinch salt
- 1 teaspoon vanilla extract
- Optional Topping: fresh herbs, flakey sea salt

Instructions

1. Preheat oven to 400°F
2. Peel and slice the sweet potatoes into 1/4 inch rounds. Add to a baking dish.

3. In a small saucepan add the butter. Heat over low heat until the butter is melted. Remove from heat.

4. Stir in the brown sugar and maple syrup.

5. Add in the spices, salt and vanilla extract, stirring to combine.

6. Carefully pour the brown sugar butter sauce over the sliced sweet potatoes. Gently stir the sweet potatoes around to coat in the butter mixture.

7. Cover the baking dish with foil and bake for 30 minutes. Stirring halfway through to ensure even baking.

8. Remove the foil and continue baking for an additional 15-30 minutes until the sweet potatoes are fork tender. Stir every 15 minutes.

9. Remove from oven and let cool at least 10 minutes to allow sauce to thicken before serving.

Prep Time: 5 Minutes

Cook Time: 25 Minutes

Servings: 10

Ingredients

- 4 ounces cream cheese, softened to room temperature
- ½ cup sour cream
- 1 16 ounce can refried beans
- 1 cup cheddar cheese, shredded, divided
- 1 cup Monterey Jack cheese, shredded, divided
- 1 4 oz can diced green chiles
- 1 packet taco seasoning, homemade taco seasoning

Optional Toppings:

- ½ cup cherry tomatoes, sliced
- 2 tbsp green onions, sliced
- 2 tbsp cilantro , chopped
- ¼ cup jalapenos, pickled
- 2 tbsp sour cream

Instructions

1. Preheat: Preheat oven to 350°F.

2. Combine Dip Ingredients: In a large bowl add the softened cream cheese and sour cream together. Stir together until well combined, might be slightly lumpy. Add in the refried beans and stir together.

3. Add in 1/2 cup of shredded cheddar cheese and 1/2 cup of shredded Monterey Jack cheese. Stir.

4. Add in the diced green chiles and taco seasoning. Stir to combine.

5. Add to Baking Dish: Spread the mixture into a 2-quart baking dish. Smooth out the top. Sprinkle with the remaining 2 cups of shredded cheese.

6. Bake: 25-30 minutes until the cheese on top is fully melted.

7. Toppings: Remove from oven and top with any optional toppings desired. Serve warm and enjoy!

Prep Time: 5 Minutes

Cook Time: 45 Minutes

Servings: 6

Ingredients

- 1 cup long grain white rice
- 2 cinnamon sticks
- 2 cloves
- ¼ tsp salt
- 4 cups whole milk
- 2 cups water
- ½ cup brown sugar
- 2 tsp vanilla

Toppings:

- Ground cinnamon
- Raisins

Instructions

1. Add rice and water in a medium size saucepan.

2. Bring to a boil, cover and reduce heat to low. Let cook for 15 minutes.

3. Remove the lid, stir the rice. Pour in the milk and add the cinnamon sticks and cloves. Stir together.

4. Increase heat to medium, stir while bringing mixture to a simmer.

5. Cover, turn to low and cook 15 minutes.

6. Remove the lid and stir in the sugar. Continue to cook an additional 15 minutes while stirring occasionally. Pudding will start to thicken.

7. Remove the pudding from the heat, stir in the vanilla extract and let sit for about 10 minutes to cool. Pudding will continue to thicken during this time.

8. Serve warm. Can also be stored in the refrigerator and served cold.

9. Top with additional sprinkles of cinnamon.

Prep Time: 6 Minutes

Cook Time: 15 Minutes

Servings: 6

Ingredients

- 2 pounds ground beef, can also use 1 pound ground beef, 1 pound ground pork
- 1/2 cup dried bread crumbs
- 1/2 onion, minced
- 4 cloves garlic, minced
- 2 tablespoons fresh parsley, diced
- 2 large eggs
- 1/4 teaspoon allspice
- 1/4 teaspoon ground nutmeg
- 2 teaspoons salt
- 1/4 teaspoon white pepper
- 1 tablespoon extra virgin olive oil

Cream Gravy:

- 2 tablespoons leftover grease from meatballs, or 2 tablespoons unsalted butter

- 1/3 cup all purpose flour
- 4 cups beef broth, unsalted
- 1 teaspoon salt
- 1/4 teaspoon white pepper
- 1 teaspoon Worcestershire, optional--advised if not using beef broth

Instructions

1. Combine the ground meats, dried bread crumbs, onion, garlic, parsley, eggs, all spice, nutmeg, salt and white pepper in a large bowl. Mix thoroughly with a stand mixer or with your hands.
2. Heat the extra virgin olive oil in a large skillet over medium heat.
3. Scoop the meat mixture using a spoon or cookie scoop. Keep the meatballs uniform in size, about 1 inch in diameter. Roll the meat between your hands to shape into a ball. Place in the skillet and cook, turning the meatballs as they cook so all sides get a sear and the meatballs cook through. To check you can cut into a meatball to ensure that no pink remains in the center. Continue until all meatballs are cooked, should take two batches to prevent overcrowding.

4. Remove the meatballs from the skillet. Drain most of the grease, keeping about 2 tablespoons.

5. Return the skillet to the stovetop. Whisk in the flour until a thick paste forms. Cook for 2-3 minutes.

6. Whisk in the beef broth. Whisk until smooth and all flour is incorporated.

7. Add salt and pepper. Whisk. Bring to a simmer.

8. Add in the meatballs and let simmer for 10 minutes.

9. Serve warm over egg noodles or mashed potatoes.

21. Baked Chicken Quesadillas

Prep Time: 10 Minutes

Cook Time: 15 Minutes

Servings: 8

Ingredients

- 2 tbsp avocado oil, can sub with vegetable, canola, or extra virgin olive oil
- 1 pound chicken, cooked and shredded
- 1 cup sour cream
- ½ tsp chili powder
- ½ tsp smoked paprika
- 1 tsp garlic powder
- 1 tsp onion powder
- ½ tsp cumin
- 1½ tsp salt
- ½ tsp ground black pepper
- 2 cup Monterey Jack cheese, shredded
- 8 flour tortillas, (6 inch size)

Toppings:

- sour cream

- pico de gallo

- guacamole

Instructions

1. Preheat oven to 425°F. Line a large baking sheet with parchment paper, brush the paper with a small amount of the oil, and set aside.
2. In a large bowl combine the shredded chicken, sour cream, and spices. Stir to combine.
3. Add the shredded cheese and mix until combined.
4. Working one tortilla at a time, spread about 1/2 cup of the chicken mixture on one half of the tortilla. Fold the tortilla over. Firmly press the tortilla together so that the top sticks to the chicken mixture in the middle (this helps with baking). Continue this process until all tortillas and chicken mixture are used.
5. Lay the folded tortillas on the prepared baking sheet. Brush the top of the tortillas with the remaining oil.
6. Bake for 15-17 minutes until tops of the tortillas are turning golden. If during the middle of baking you see that the tortillas are bending up, carefully press them back down using a spoon or spatula.

Prep Time: 10 Minutes

Cook Time: 30 Minutes

Servings: 6

Ingredients

- 1 lb ground beef
- ½ cup onion, diced
- 1 green bell pepper, diced
- 2 cups potato, peeled and diced
- 4 cloves garlic, minced
- 8 ounces tomato sauce
- 1½ cup beef broth
- 1 tsp salt
- ¼ tsp ground black pepper
- 1 tsp ground cumin
- 1 tsp ground coriander
- 1 bay leaf

Instructions

1. Heat a large skillet over medium heat, add ground beef. Cook over medium heat while breaking up the meat. Cook until mostly browned, drain grease and return to heat.

2. Add in diced onion, green bell pepper and potatoes. Continue to cook over medium heat until onion and peppers are softened. Add garlic and cook an additional 30 seconds.

3. Pour in tomato sauce and beef broth. Add in seasonings: salt, pepper, cumin, and coriander. Stir to combine. Add bay leaf.

4. Bring mixture to a simmer, cover and let cook for 10 minutes.

5. Remove lid, stir, and continue cooking with the lid off for an additional 10 minutes or until potatoes are softened and most of the liquid is gone.

6. Serve warm with flour tortillas and rice.

Prep Time: 15 Minutes

Cook Time: 0 Minutes

Servings: 6

Ingredients

Avocado Summer Rolls:

- Rice Paper Wrappers
- 1 cup Baby Spinach
- 1 cup Bean Sprouts
- 1 Orange Bell Pepper
- 1 Yellow Bell Pepper
- 1 Carrots, grated
- 1 Avocado, sliced

Sweet 'N Spicy Cilantro Dipping Sauce:

- 1/2 cup cilantro leaves, packed
- 1/3 cup extra virgin olive oil
- 1/3 cup agave
- 1/2 tbsp white vinegar

- 1½ tbsp Chili Garlic Sauce

Instructions

Avocado Summer Rolls

1. Prepare all the veggies, slice the bell peppers and avocado, set aside.
2. Fill a large dish, or pan with room temperature water. Dip one rice paper into the water, ensure that the entire paper is submerged into the water. Only leave it in the water for about 5 seconds. Place the wet rice paper onto a hard surface. Set filling, minus the avocado, on top of the paper, off to one side. Next to the filling, set two to three slices of avocado.
3. Start rolling the papers from the side closest to the fillings. Roll the fillings in first, then another roll to capture the avocado (this is how you make the avocado show on the top). Fold in both sides, and continue rolling, this will completely enclose the filling into the rice paper. Set aside and repeat with the remaining papers.

Sweet 'N Spicy Cilantro Dipping Sauce

1. Add the ingredients into a food processor, process together for about 1 minute, until the cilantro is completely chopped up and all ingredients are mixed together.
2. Spoon sauce into a serving bowl.
3. Serve immediately and enjoy!

Prep Time: 15 Minutes

Cook Time: 3hrs 30 Minutes

Servings: 6

Ingredients

- 3 pounds sweet potato, about 3 large sweet potatoes
- 1 cup water
- 1/2 cup light brown sugar
- 1/4 cup butter
- 1/4 teaspoon cinnamon
- 1/4 teaspoon nutmeg
- 2 large eggs
- 1/2 cup whole milk

Topping:

- 1 cup pecan halves, roughly chopped
- 2/3 cup light brown sugar
- 1/4 cup all purpose flour
- 1 teaspoon vanilla extract
- 1/3 cup butter melted

Instructions

1. Peel and chop the sweet potatoes. Add to slow cooker with the 1 cup of water. Cook on high heat for 3 hours until the sweet potatoes are softened.
2. Add the light brown sugar, butter, cinnamon, nutmeg, eggs, and whole milk. Mash the potatoes and mix with all the ingredients until smooth.
3. In a small mixing bowl combine the ingredients for the topping. Stir to combine. Spoon onto the top of the sweet potatoes. Cover and continue cooking on high for another 30 minutes.
4. Allow to cool for 10 minutes to help set and thicken.
5. Serve warm and enjoy!

Prep Time: 30 Minutes

Cook Time: 30 Minutes

Servings: 10

Ingredients

- 6 tbsp unsalted butter
- 1 cup yellow onion, diced
- 1 red bell pepper, diced
- 1 green bell pepper, diced
- 3 cloves garlic, minced
- 1 tsp ground cumin
- 1 tbsp chili powder
- 1 tsp salt
- ½ tsp black pepper
- ¼ cup all purpose flour
- 1¾ cup chicken broth
- 1 (10 ounce) diced tomatoes with green chiles, drained
- 1½ cup sour cream
- 2 lbs chicken, cooked and shredded
- 4 cups monterey jack cheese, shredded
- 18 corn tortillas, yellow or white

- ¼ cup canola oil

Optional Toppings:

- cilantro, chopped
- sour cream

Instructions

1. Preheat oven to 350°F degrees. Spray 3 quart baking dish with cooking spray and set aside.
2. In a large skillet over medium heat melt the butter. Once melted add the onion, and bell peppers. Allow to cook for several minutes, stirring occasionally, until tender and browned.
3. Add in the garlic, cumin, chili powder, salt, and black pepper. Stir to coat the veggies in the seasonings.
4. Sprinkle the flour into the skillet. Stir to coat the veggies in the flour, will end up with a thick paste. Cook briefly for 2-3 minutes.
5. Pour in the broth and stir. Bring mixture to a boil while stirring and let simmer while stirring for about 2-3 minutes until thick. Remove from heat, allow to cool for about 2 minutes and stir in the diced tomatoes with green chiles and the sour cream. Stir to

combine. Add the shredded chicken and stir until mixed. Set aside.

6. Pour the canola oil into a large skillet and heat over medium heat. Once the oil is heated carefully lay the tortillas in the oil in batches. Cook until just lightly fried, they should be flexible still and not crispy. Remove from oil and place onto a plate lined with paper towels to catch the remaining oil.

7. Once all tortillas are cooked layer 6 tortillas on the bottom of the baking dish. Layer the tortillas to cover as much of the dish as possible. Top with half of the chicken mixture then one third of the cheese. Repeat by layering 6 more tortillas, the remaining half of the chicken mixture, and one third of the cheese. Top with the remaining tortillas and the rest of the cheese.

8. Cover the baking dish with foil and bake for 15 minutes. Remove the foil and continue baking for an additional 10 minutes. Remove from the oven allow to cool for several minutes then serve warm. Can serve with additional sour cream and fresh cilantro.

Prep Time: 5 Minutes

Cook Time: 10 Minutes

Servings: 6

Ingredients

- 2 cups chicken broth , unsalted
- 2 cups milk
- ½ teaspoon salt
- 1 cup quick grits, or substitute with other grits just read above to be able to adjust cooking time
- 1/4 cup unsalted butter
- 1 cup sharp cheddar cheese, shredded

Topping:

- pads of butter
- black pepper
- extra shredded cheese

Instructions

1. Combine the chicken broth and milk in a medium size saucepan. Heat over medium heat. Bring to a simmer.

2. Stir in the salt. Then add the grits slowly while stirring. Stir until all grits are well mixed.

3. Cover and reduce heat to low for 3-4 minutes. Remove the lid and stir the grits. Continue stirring while cooking over low for an additional 1-2 minutes. The grits will be tender when done cooking.

4. Turn the heat off. Add in the butter and cheese. Stir until well mixed.

5. Serve immediately. Top with additional shredded cheese, butter and fresh pepper if desired.

Prep Time: 10 Minutes

Cook Time: 20 Minutes

Servings: 8

Ingredients

- 4 strips bacon
- 1/2 cup onion, diced
- 3 cloves garlic, minced
- 2 tbsp all purpose flour
- 32 ounces corn, frozen or canned (approx 9 ears of corn)
- 1 lb gold potatoes, diced 1/2 inch cubes
- 2 tsp salt
- ¼ tsp ground black pepper
- ¼ tsp paprika
- 4 cups chicken broth, unsalted
- 1 cup half and half, (or milk of preference)
- 1 lb ham, diced into 1/2 inch cubes

Instructions

1. In a large dutch oven or pot, cook the bacon until desired crispness, remove the bacon from the pot and set aside, keep 2 tbsp of grease, drain any excess.
2. Add the diced onion and cook until softened and translucent. Add the garlic and cook an additional 30 seconds.
3. Stir in the flour, allow this to cook for 1-2 minutes.
4. Stir in the salt, pepper, and paprika. Pour in the chicken broth. Stir to combine.
5. Add in the diced potatoes. Bring to a low simmer. Cover and cook for 10-15 minutes over medium heat.
6. Remove the lid, add in the corn and continue to cook for an additional 10 minutes until the corn is heated through and the potatoes are fork tender.
7. Turn off the heat and using an immersion blender blend up the soup to desired consistency. Be sure to leave some chunks of potato and corn in the soup. The more you blend the thicker the soup will be. IF you don't have an immersion blender, remove a portion of the soup carefully and blend in a blender or food processor. Then return to the pot.

8. Optional: sear the ham in a skillet over medium high heat for 5 minutes, turning to ensure all sides are seared.

9. Add the ham to the pot and the cooked diced bacon, setting some aside for garnishing. Stir to combine. If you skipped searing the ham, you will need to turn the heat back on under the soup pot to give the ham time to warm in the soup before moving on.

10. With the heat still off the pot, stir in the half and half.

11. Serve soup warm with a garnish of fresh chives or parsley, fresh ground pepper, and cooked bacon.

Prep Time: 5 Minutes

Cook Time: 25 Minutes

Servings: 4

Ingredients

- 4 slices bacon
- 1 stalk celery, chopped
- ½ cup onion, diced
- 1 bell pepper, seeds removed, diced
- 2 cloves garlic, minced
- ¼ cup all purpose flour
- 1 (12 ounce) beer
- 1½ cups chicken broth
- 1 cup heavy cream
- 8 ounces sharp cheddar cheese, shredded
- ½ tsp paprika
- salt & pepper, to taste

Instructions

1. Cook the bacon in a large dutch oven or stock pot over medium-high heat. Cook the bacon to desired crispness. Remove the bacon and leave the grease.
2. Add the celery, onion, and bell pepper. Stir while sautéing for about 5 minutes until the veggies are tender and the onion is translucent. Add in the garlic and cook an additional 30 seconds.
3. Add the flour and stir until the vegetables are coated in the flour. Cook for 2-3 minutes.
4. Add the beer, chicken broth and heavy cream. Stir until fully combined. Bring to a boil then lower the heat to medium.
5. Continue to cook for another 15 minutes.
6. Remove the pot from the heat and stir in the sharp cheddar cheese. Stir while the cheese melts.
7. Add the paprika. Add the salt and pepper to taste.
8. Serve soup warm garnished with parsley, more shredded sharp cheddar cheese and crumbled bacon on the top.

Prep Time: 15 Minutes

Cook Time: 30 Minutes

Servings: 6

Ingredients

- 3 pounds apples , peeled, cored, sliced (favorites include Honeycrisp, Gala, and Granny Smith)
- 1/2 cup light brown sugar
- 2 tsp ground cinnamon
- 1/2 tsp ground nutmeg
- 1/4 tsp ground cloves
- 1/8 tsp salt
- juice from 1/2 a lemon
- 1 tsp vanilla extract
- 2 tbsp unsalted butter

Instructions

1. Preheat: Preheat the oven to 350°F degrees.
2. Prepare Apples: Peel the apples, cut and remove the core and cut into slices about 1/3-1/2 an inch thick.

3. Combine Ingredients: Add the apples to a large bowl or you can mix right in a pie dish, or 2 quart baking dish. Add the light brown sugar, cinnamon, nutmeg, cloves, salt, lemon juice and vanilla extract. Stir to combine. If using a bowl, spoon the apples into a pie dish or 2 quart baking dish.

4. Butter: Cut the butter into small squares, and place them over the top of the apples.

5. Baking: Bake for 30 minutes, stirring after the apples have baked for 15 minutes. This prevents apples on the top from drying. Bake until the apples are tender and soft.

6. Serve: Remove and serve with a scoop of vanilla ice cream on top. Serve warm.

Prep Time: 10 Minutes

Cook Time: 20 Minutes

Servings: 6

Ingredients

- 2 lbs baby red potatoes
- 1 tsp course sea salt
- 6 slices bacon, cooked & crumbled
- 5 ounces blue cheese
- ½ cup green onion, sliced
- ¼ cup mayonnaise
- ¼ cup sour cream
- ½ tsp dill
- ¼ tsp salt
- ¼ tsp ground mustard
- ½ tsp onion powder

Instructions

1. Chop the baby red potatoes into small 1 inch cubes, place into a large pot and cover with water. Bring to a

boil and add the coarse sea salt. Boil for approximately 15-20 minutes, or until the potatoes are soft and tender and able to be mashed with a fork.

2. Remove the pot from the heat and pour the potatoes into a strainer to drain out all the water. Place potatoes into a large bowl and allow to cool to room temperature, or place into the refrigerator to cool down.

3. In a small bowl combine the mayonnaise, sour cream, dill, salt, ground mustard, and onion powder. Stir to combine.

4. Add the bacon, blue cheese and green onion to the cooled potatoes.

5. Spoon dressing over the top of the salad and stir to combine. Cover and chill for at least 30 minutes before serving.